Inky, My Dad & Me

by Kym Motley

Printed in the United States of America

First Printing, 2013

ISBN 978-0-9910884-1-6

Kym Motley

www.kymmotley.com

For Inky, my teacher

For Dad, my inspiration

And for all of my guardian angels, thank you

Table of Contents

Preface

My dad used to tell this joke about a guy who was lost and called a friend for directions. He said, "I'm at the corner of Walk and Don't Walk." Obviously, the guy didn't look up to read the name of the streets, just the traffic signal directly in front of him. When I think about why I wanted to write this book, this joke came to mind. Several friends have asked me for advice regarding their dying loved ones, and all of them started at this intersection. Walk and Don't Walk could be the corner of chemo and hospice, denial and acceptance, or any other combination of circumstances and mixed emotions. Here, I will share practical advice for friends and caregivers of dying loved ones through my experiences with my kitty, Inky, and my dad.

A couple months before my father was diagnosed with pancreatic cancer, my beloved black, Burmese kitty, Inky, was diagnosed with cancer. This came as a complete shock. Unlike my asthmatic, orange tabby cat, Stinky, Inky was never sick. Through his diagnosis, treatment, and ultimate passing, Inky was my teacher. I had the displeasure of losing Inky and my dad within six months of each other; however, Inky showed me how to be fully present and loving for my dad as he walked with death.

My father's third bout with cancer brought with it a dark cloud of despair. His first two battles were of the Non-Hodgkin's Lymphoma variety, and they came with an 80% chance of recovery. Determined to beat the disease, my dad fought the first two rounds and won. Despite his victory, he said, "If the cancer comes back, I'm not doing chemo. It's like going to hell and back." I knew he meant it. He also said he spent his time waiting for the other shoe to drop. I tried not to think about it, but the shoe dropped seven years later, and although I remembered what my dad said, we were not prepared for the arduous road ahead.

I did know one thing – I loved my father very, very much. Although I, too, was scared, I told him, "I'm going to hold your hand and drop you off at the pearly gates." He replied, "I know." It's at this intersection of fear and love my journey began. By becoming friends with death, I also became friends with life. I found peace about my dad's impending death and embraced the future I wanted to create for myself. The journey from the corner of Walk and Don't Walk is different for everyone. I hope that by sharing my experience I can help others find peace in their journeys with their loved ones and within themselves.

1

Find Your Loved Ones and Meet Them There

Inky

It was 2009, between Thanksgiving and Christmas. As I played with Inky one afternoon, I felt a hard lump on his right hind foot. The lump was half the size of a golf ball, and it didn't move. My heart sank. I scheduled a vet visit and cried uncontrollably. The next day, the vet performed a biopsy, and then we waited for pathology to provide the lab results. Three days later, Inky was diagnosed with lymphoma. My vet did not recommend chemotherapy, but she asked if I wanted to see a specialist. Still in denial and determined to beat the disease, I asked for the referral. The following week, we began the routine of weekly oncology visits — blood tests, chemotherapy, and appetite stimulants.

My Dad

In January 2010, my parents went to a routine doctor visit, and the first inclinations that my dad had cancer again were revealed. We were referred to a specialist for a biopsy. My parents and I waited anxiously for the test results. A week later, my dad was diagnosed with pancreatic cancer. My heart sank again. After my dad's diagnosis, I accompanied my parents to their oncologist appointment. We were on a first-name basis with the doctor by this time, and all of us agreed that it was a bittersweet reunion. My supporting role was somewhere between courtroom transcriber and Philadelphia lawyer. I copiously scribbled conversations verbatim and asked questions on behalf of my parents. My dad inquired about surgery. Not an option. He then asked about chemotherapy. The oncologist told him it was an option, so my dad decided to do chemo. He excused my dad from the room and had a follow-up conversation with my mom and me. "I cannot save him this time, but the chemo will buy him some time. Your dad is a fighter – as long as he wants to fight, we can do the chemo. When he becomes tired, we'll stop." Although the record showed my dad's reticence to undergo chemo a third time, he was sitting in front of me signing up for treatment. My mom acknowledged the doctor's comments with continuous head nods, but I knew the info was too much for her to process. Looking at the signs, Mom was in shock, Dad was in denial, and I was reluctantly realistic.

I quickly realized "getting everyone on the same page" would be a fruitless endeavor. This was not something that could be solved with a PowerPoint deck in an hour meeting. I decided to meet my mom and dad where they were, which meant not talking my dad out of chemo.

What you can do…

If you are a caregiver, offer to go to a doctor appointment. Just your presence in the room can provide comfort and confidence. Actively listen, take notes, and ask questions in a considerate manner. If you have a question that doesn't seem appropriate to ask in front of your loved one, ask to see the oncologist or nurse afterwards.

If you are friends with a caregiver, offer to meet your friend for coffee and conversation. Active listening is all that's required – no advice is necessary, unless solicited.

2

Listen Intently, With Your Eyes, Ears and Heart

Release Me

For weeks, I dropped Inky off at the kitty oncologist on Tuesdays. We left the house at 7:15 am, and upon arrival at the specialist's office we waited patiently to hear our name called. The lobby was bright, white, and medicinal in nature; however, it felt like we were in a William Blake painting of purgatory. Other pet parents waited with trepidation. I could tell by the other animals' shaved bellies and bandages their pet parents were also hoping for a cure for some incorrigible disease. When the vet technician called Inky's name, I gave her the rundown on the past week — whether he was eating and pooping, if he was in pain, and whether he emitted a strange smell. The technician copiously jotted down my comments each week and took Inky.

I cried in the car on the way to work and waited in anticipation for the vet's report around lunchtime. His blood count determined whether he would receive chemotherapy. Quite often, the vet reported, "Inky is doing fantastic. He is responding well to treatment." His tumor was shrinking, and it validated my valiant efforts to save him. He was not dying on my watch; no way. After every visit, I thought, "We beat cancer for another week."

After several weeks of the tumor shrinking, Inky's tumor began to grow aggressively. I talked with the oncologist, and her recommendation was to treat Inky with radiation for five days, then return to chemotherapy. Radiation was estimated at $500 a day, and travel to a neighboring state would have been required. I was faced with finding a pet-friendly hotel, working remotely, and subjecting my Inky to five days of hell in an unknown location. I began to contemplate whether fighting cancer was the answer. Although Inky had responded well to the treatment for three months, he was becoming very tired and poopy. Conventional medicine had worn out its welcome, so I decided to find a pet medium to talk to Inky.

I gave the medium a quick description of Inky – a black Burmese kitty with big yellow eyes. "I've got him, she said."

She was instantly amazed at Inky's spirit, which she described as very evolved and insightful. This was in alignment with how others described him. One of my friends referred to him as Buddha Kitty. I asked Inky how he felt about continuing with chemotherapy. He said, "I see your valiant efforts to save me, and sometimes I want to continue, and sometimes I want to stop. I know you love me, but you cannot save me. Are you ready to release me from this treatment?" His words hung in the air. If I loved Inky, I needed to honor his request. I did, after all, want to find out how he was feeling. My voice was full of fear and sadness when I told him, "Yes, I will honor your request and release you from treatment." Inky continued, "I want to live a clean life – I want to spend time with you without the toxins in my body. I want to be fully present for the time I have left, and I want you to be fully present with me." I did not anticipate learning my biggest life lesson during this session. Little did I know, both of my kitties were terribly insightful and aware of what was going on with my dad and me.

I adopted Inky at the age of two, and for nine of the eleven years he was with me, he hardly meowed. He saved a few sacred hisses for his brother, Stinky, an orange tabby cat and master antagonist. I asked Inky why he recently started meowing. "I had to get your attention. You've been in a rut when you come home from your workaday." This was also true. I had not been happy with work and was on autopilot. Next, I described Stinky to the medium. "He's an orange tabby…." "Oh, I've got him…he's been listening to the conversation," she said. She laughed when Stinky told her, "I don't smell, I'm very clean. It's my personality." She described Stinky as having a joker-like persona. Yes, right again – Stinky is always looking for things to get into and knows which buttons to push when he doesn't get what he wants. Stinky is fearless, has alpha male tendencies, and thinks the world rotates around him. And it did, until Inky got sick. "I've known about this from the beginning," Stinky informed me in his "know-it-all" fashion. I noticed whenever Inky felt bad, Stinky curled up next to him. It didn't matter if Inky had that "I just came back from the vet smell," Stinky was always comforting his brother. I also witnessed Stinky listening to Inky with his heart by stepping down from his position as alpha male. He ceded his primo spot in the bed and allowed Inky to curl up next to my chest at night. Inky no longer asked for permission to cuddle. Stinky manned his new nighttime station at the bottom of the bed and watched over us. At night, I could feel Inky's purr next to my heart. It put me at ease, for in that moment, everything was ok.

Whites of Your Eyeballs

I called my mom and dad every day like clockwork. I could tell by my mother's tone, not her words, how they were doing. The answer was always, "Everything's fine." However, I knew better. I had to see for myself. As I came through the door and said my hellos, my mom would sometimes say, "You didn't have to come over – we talked to you on the phone. We're doing ok." I replied, "Well, I just wanted to see the whites of your eyeballs." It became a running joke with my parents, and whenever I talked to my dad on the phone, I said, "I'm calling to see the whites of your eyeballs." He replied, "Can you hear them?" or "They're white…just like they were yesterday."

I had a candid conversation with my dad one evening about his illness. He said, "Y'know, you're joking about seeing the whites of my eyeballs, but I know the cancer is progressing when my eyes turn yellow." He was referring to jaundice, which would eventually set in as part of pancreatic cancer. Seven years ago, he was able to withstand the toxic cocktails and side effects – standing firmly, like the 60-year oak tree that still stands in my parents' front yard. At 84, my dad was older and more fragile. He realized prolonging his life didn't necessarily mean his quality of life would improve significantly. He and my mother decided to stop treatment.

During a later visit, I overheard my dad on the phone with a distant relative asking for pain medicine. "Have you been back to the doctor?" I asked my mom. "Ask your father about it," she replied. I asked my dad whether he and my mother went to the follow-up appointment at the oncologist. "No, and I'm not going back to the doctor. I don't want any more chemo. I don't want to be poked. I don't want fluids. Do you know what it's like to sit in a room filled with people getting chemo?" I thought about the sitting area in the back room – a semicircle of La-Z-Boy chairs. When filled, I could only imagine the heavy cloud of morosity looming over the patients as they sat for hours with an IV pumping chemicals through their veins.

Unbeknownst to my parents, I had already been down this road with Inky. I understood why they decided not to continue with treatment. I also knew this meant death was imminent. I had to convince my parents to go back to the doctor one last time so my dad could be referred to Hospice. "He has to see the whites of your eyeballs. You have to go back one last time." Begrudgingly, my dad agreed to go back to the oncologist.

What you can do…

If you are a caregiver, just listen. Listening creates a safe place for your loved one to be honest, and it shows you're there for support. Listening with your eyes means being observant. Does what your loved one says match what you see? Listening with your ears and heart means not always filling the awkward moments of silence with mindless chatter. Sometimes, silently reading a book or watching a movie with your loved one is all that's needed. Take cues from your loved one. If s/he feels like talking about the illness, s/he will do so. If s/he feels like talking about the small stuff, share news about your new outfit or the award you recently won. It will remind your loved one that s/he is an important part of your life and still part of this world. Try not to take any emotions you encounter — anger, denial, depression — personally.

If you are friends with a caregiver, just listen, listen, and listen some more. You can also listen with your eyes and heart by watching your friend's actions. If your friend is becoming consumed with caregiving, offer to help research options for support. So many services are available, but when you're close to terminal illness, it's difficult to see options available to you.

In addition to emotional consumption, caregiving is time consuming and physically demanding. If your friend is checking on loved ones before and after work, offer to cook a meal or run an errand.

3

Send Love, No Matter What

A Change of Heart

The day of our oncologist visit for the Hospice referral, my mom called and said, "Your dad changed his mind. Tell the doctor we're not coming." I asked to speak to him, knowing he was going to blast me. My dad fussed – the phone felt hot with anger, fear, and frustration. I let him finish, and then in a calm tone I asked, "Haven't I always been in your corner? I understand why you don't want to continue with treatment. I promise no one will poke you anymore or make you take fluids. The doctor will understand your decision and help you manage the pain. I'll be there at 1:30 tomorrow to pick you up."

During the visit, the doctor explained he was referring my dad to Hospice. He confirmed for my dad there would be no more chemotherapy, no more poking and prodding, and that the goal of Hospice care was to keep him comfortable. As we left the doctor's office, my dad put his arm around me and said, "I was so mad at you yesterday, but you took care of me." I smiled at my dad and helped him into the car.

My mom and my four older brothers were all at different intersections in their grief. I tried desperately to get them to meet me at my dad's corner, but my message was rebuffed, leaving me feeling angry and isolated. I called the pet medium again to talk with Inky. I asked him how to deal with these feelings. "Send them love – they can't fight love," he said. Inky explained that my mom was very scared and her anger stemmed from the fear of losing her beloved husband of 60 years. We were all on the same journey but we took different paths — some longer some shorter — with different stops along the way.

What you can do…

If you are a caregiver, send love no matter what. Make the conscious choice to act out of love instead of fear. Your loved one will need love while finding peace with death. Send your family members love, too. They will go through the phases of grief at different paces and in different ways. Judgment about whether their paths are too short or too long, right or wrong, healthy or unhealthy will drain your energy and cause friction. If, however, you feel your loved one is in danger, make the doctors aware and ask for help in maintaining a safe environment. After you lose a loved one, the family dynamic is never the same. Find peace in knowing you did not drain your much-needed energy on negative actions or feelings.

If you are friends with a caregiver, send love, too. Help recharge your friend's batteries so s/he can show up and send love to her/his dying loved one. Caregiving is an "around the clock" activity, and schedules are unpredictable. Although your friend may not be able to talk every time you call, it is comforting to read or hear a message and know someone is sending you good thoughts.

4

Be Open to Hospice, Your New Best Friend

How Much Time Does He Have?

After Inky's treatments were over, I went back to my vet to see how to keep him comfortable. "How much time does he have?" I asked. My vet very lovingly told me, "You will know." The new responsibility of knowing when to put Inky down was overwhelming. What if I did it too early? What if I did it too late? What if he was in pain and I didn't know it? *How will I know?*

The vet sent me home with appetite stimulants and liquid pain medication pre-drawn in vials. Chemotherapy visits were replaced with weekly check-ins for kitty acupuncture to help manage the pain, a weight check, and a once over. I didn't know what tomorrow would bring, but I had faith in knowing I was not alone in my journey with Inky. Somehow, I would know when it was time for my dear kitty to make his transition.

Blankets Change Things

I visited my dad on a not-so-good day. Consternation was written all over his face – furrowed brow, eyes closed, head down. When I asked him if there was anything I could do, he shook his head, "No." He said, "I knew this pain was going to get me – get to the point where it wouldn't go away." "Do you need a pain pill?" I asked. He nodded his head, "Yes." Unable to leave my dad in pain, I waited for the Oxycontin to take effect. Ten minutes later, the pain started to subside. Before I left, I asked my dad if he wanted his blanket. He nodded his head, "Yes." I grabbed the blanket and covered his legs and feet. The burgundy and forest green throw blanket was quite pedestrian – there was no story or special event attached to it; however, it was my dad's armor against cancer. The blanket represented the not-so-distant memory of having no pain – of resting on the floor reading a golf magazine, listening to classical music, and helping my mom with the crossword puzzle.

Being under the care of Hospice is like being in an exclusive club no one talks about and therefore is often misunderstood. My dad thought Hospice was keeping him alive; my mom thought Hospice was killing him. When your loved one is terminally ill, you have access to a myriad of services. Hospice helps your loved one stay comfortable and maintain dignity, and it provides support for your family members.

My first Hospice session was with a counselor who met with me to determine where I was in the grief process. Afterwards, she assigned a social worker to me. The social worker became my lifeline. We talked about my dad's pain, how my family was coping, and how I was feeling as one of the primary caregivers. At the end of my session, she gave me a pink and green crocheted blanket. On the front was a note attached with a pin in the shape of a cross. A group of ladies at a nearby Presbyterian church had made the prayer blanket for someone who needed comfort. It didn't matter I was Unitarian and the blanket was of Presbyterian descent. I knew prayer, in any religion, was about connecting with others. At that moment, I felt connected — I was no longer alone in my struggle to get through my dad's illness. Thanks to the ladies at the Presbyterian church, I now had a special blanket to comfort me.

The New Normal

My dad's Hospice routine included visits from his head nurse every other day. She took his vitals, refilled a pillbox the size of an iPad, and talked with me about my dad's progression. Also in rotation were home health aids that came to bathe him, change diapers and bandages, trim his hair, and shape up his mustache. After one visit, I grabbed the mirror and said, "You still look handsome, Dad." He took a look at his clean shaven face and his navy blue plaid pajamas and said, "I sure do, don't I?" My dad's sense of pride and dignity eclipsed the notion he was now bedridden and growing weary.

No one really knew how much time my dad had left in this lifetime; I knew this from my experience with Inky. Unlike Corporate America, Project Pearly Gates was not adhering to a schedule, and there was very little way to know what would happen next. I continued to stay in the moment and be available for my dad. Whatever happened, we were in it together.

What you can do…

If you are a caregiver, be open to Hospice. This is a crucial point in your loved one's journey. Acceptance of Hospice gives your loved one the opportunity to make the transition with comfort and dignity. Based on your loved one's wishes and your physical, emotional, and financial capabilities, you can choose to take care of your loved one at home, or you can admit your loved one to a Hospice house.

Ask yourself the following questions:

1. Does your loved one have a preference for staying home vs. being in a medical facility?

2. Are you able to share shifts with family members or close friends to take care of your loved one?

3. Are you physically able to lift and move your loved one?

4. How do you feel about changes in your home? Are you open to receiving visitors, medical staff, and medical supplies?

5. Do bodily fluids, diapers, or bedsores make you squeamish?

6. If you have health insurance, are you able to take time off from work under the Family Medical Leave Act (FMLA)?

7. If you are not eligible for FMLA, do you have a nest egg for living expenses and incidentals?

8. Does your loved one have a life insurance policy? Keep in mind a few expenses are not covered by your loved one's life insurance policy, such as printing an obituary in the local newspaper.

If you choose to take care of your loved one at home, be prepared for your environment to change. Your loved one will require care 24 hours a day. The house will be peppered with diapers, ointment, and medications, and a Do Not Resuscitate (DNR) order will be displayed prominently in your home. Eventually, you may need a portable toilet and a hospital bed. The nurses will show you their techniques for lifting and moving your loved one, which takes some muscle. If you are able to share shifts with others, do so to prevent physical fatigue and emotional exhaustion. At a minimum, have someone to relieve you for a little bit each day.

If you choose a Hospice house, your loved one will receive around the clock care. Hospice houses are usually peaceful, flower-filled settings. The staff is kind, courteous, and patient. Rooms have space for you to take a nap or spend the night, if you so choose.

In addition to medical assistance, Hospice provides a plethora of supplemental services. Choose a pampered service to help your loved one feel handsome or beautiful, such as a clean shave or a manicure. Does your loved one have a story to tell? If so, Hospice will help record it. There is nothing like hearing your loved one's voice after she or he has made the transition. Depending on the time of your loved one's passing, Hospice will also arrange for holiday meals, such as Thanksgiving dinner.

Recharge your batteries so you don't take your frustration out on your loved one. Although unintended, sometimes abuse occurs. Hospice offers individual and group therapy for family members. Fight your feelings of reluctance and take advantage of the counseling services. Provide yourself with a safe place to vent your frustrations, share your concerns, and learn from others' experiences.

If you're friends with a caregiver, meet your friend for coffee or a walk. Time outside of the caregiving routine is critical for your friend to feel re-energized. Visits are welcome, but don't create additional work. If you bring a meal, make it easy to eat and clean up. If you're so inclined, help out with housework or errands.

5

Ask For and Accept Help

Help Doesn't Have To Be A Four-Letter Word

Before ending Inky's chemotherapy, my Tuesday routine of driving to the oncologist, heading to work, driving back to the vet on my lunch hour, taking Inky home, and then going back to work got mentally and physically exhausting. My friend's son offered to pick Inky up on Tuesdays and take him home for me. At first, I proclaimed, "No, I signed up for this so it's my responsibility to get him to the doctor and home." A couple weeks later, after exhaustion set in, my friend's mother lamented, "People love you, and they want to help. Let them help you." I finally accepted his offer to help. Every Tuesday, I dropped Inky off, and every Tuesday, my friend's son took Inky home. Each week, he called me at work and said, "He's safe and sound, Kym." I let out a sigh of relief.

The head nurse set up shop in my mom's nerve center, the kitchen table. Out of her black bag came pills, a stethoscope, and a plethora of supplies – diapers, bandages, and ointment. From my mom's point of view, the sacred space that provided an escape from chemo treatments and hospital visits had been turned into a military operation. I moved in to my old room and strategically placed baby monitors throughout the house. "Wherever you are, Dad, I can hear you. Just say my name, and I'll be there." My dad sighed with relief while my mother was still digesting the recent home invasion.

All You Have To Do Is Ask

My dad's head nurse gave me the rundown on how to dispense medications, change diapers, and redress bedsore wounds. I knew panicking would not make my mom or dad feel better, but I was secretly having a meltdown. I talked with my oldest niece later that afternoon. "I don't know how I'm going to change diapers or redress bedsore wounds," I said. She replied, "Let me call my grandma. She knows about home health." I held my breath as she made the call. "She's on her way," she said.

My niece's grandmother had her grandson in tow. He was also well-versed in home health care. Upon arrival, they asked for new sheets, a new diaper, pajamas, a washcloth, warm water, and soap. My mom drew water in a basin while I grabbed the sheets, diaper, and pajamas. With little fuss, they changed the sheets with my dad in the bed, similar to a magician pulling the tablecloth off the table without knocking over the setting. Next, they gave my dad a bath, changed his diaper, and put on a fresh pair of pajamas. I was awestruck by the ease with which they worked their magic. I was equally overwhelmed by their unconditional love. Taking care of my dad was not on their agenda that evening, yet they dropped everything to help us. My niece's grandma reminded me God was looking out for us. "It's going to be ok. You call me if you need anything," she said. Hearing her voice reminded me help is there when you need it. All you have to do is ask. Let God, or the Universe, figure out the rest.

A few days later, one of my best friends organized a food tree. She coordinated drop off locations, and casseroles, soup, and salads came in abundance. I could tell my mom was a bit hesitant by her quizzical response, "People bring food after someone has died, not before." I echoed my friend's words, "People love us, and they want to help, Mom. Let them help."

It was healing to eat healthy food prepared with love from friends. It took mental and physical exhaustion for me to understand I wasn't supposed to do everything myself. By allowing others to help, I allowed them to show me love. By accepting love, I created connection and community with others.

What you can do…

If you are a caregiver, don't be afraid to ask for help. Don't hesitate to call the Hospice line if you have questions of any kind. They are available 24/7. Remember, there's no such thing as a stupid question when you're taking care of a dying loved one.

Your friends and family want to help, but they may not know what to do. Make a list of house chores, errands, and food preferences. Enlist a close friend or two to help with organizing so you don't get overwhelmed. Let that person know what you need, and empower him or her to coordinate with others on your behalf. Help will come from unexpected people and places — it will pleasantly surprise you.

If you are friends with a caregiver, ask how you can help. If you are unable to perform a task, do you know someone else who can help? Perhaps your cousin has an extra walker or a pillow wedge for the bed. Most importantly, listen with your eyes, ears, and heart, and then you will know what to do.

6

The Final Days

The Knowing

The last two nights before Inky died, he refused to sleep upstairs with Stinky and me. We joined him downstairs on the sofa, and I knew his time was drawing near. Those two days were filled with more frequent pain medication, and on that third day, the twinkle was gone from Inky's eyes. I called my vet and told her it was time. She made an appointment for 7pm that evening to come to the house. I spent the afternoon outside with Inky taking photos, eating rotisserie chicken, and letting him explore the neighborhood.

The vet arrived with snacks, a towel, and an IV. She gave Inky a Fancy Feast appetizer, which he ate heartily. I then held him in my arms. After a few minutes, she asked, "Are you ready?" I reluctantly yet bravely answered, "Yes." She inserted an IV, gave Inky medication, and within minutes, his spirit left his body.

As I held him in my arms, I was grateful. Grateful for the lessons he taught me about being fully present. Grateful for the insight he gave me regarding my father's "turning," as he called it. Grateful for reminding me to send love no matter what. The huge spirit contained in his little 12-pound cat package humbled me. I was honored to be Inky's beloved companion in this lifetime.

The Turning

My dad's world got smaller during his last 10 days. Just as his world moved from outside to inside, and from inside to the bedroom, his body followed a similar pattern. He grew too weary to sit up in bed and spent most of the day sleeping. The head nurse explained the science behind my dad's turning. Unlike before when she could not tell me how much time my dad had left, the body shows telltale signs when it is in the final stages of life. My dad's body slowed its production of saliva, which caused his faint whisper. His circulation no longer provided blood to his extremities, which turned the soles of his feet blue. His kidneys began to shut down, which caused his urine to turn reddish-brown. I frequently swabbed his mouth with water-saturated sponges to moisten his mouth. I checked his feet several times daily to make sure they were propped up by a rolled towel to prevent bedsores. The myriad of pills were replaced with liquid morphine to keep him comfortable. I reminded myself my dad was still in there. Although his physical world was getting smaller, he could still hear, feel, think, and love.

The morning of my dad's last day, the head nurse asked me to let the family know they needed to see my dad pronto. Our Hospice counselor met with interested family members for pre-death counseling. I sat with my dad for several hours that day and held his hand. It was warm and soft. He tossed and turned. "Are you going to roll out of the bed on my watch?" I asked. Although he couldn't talk, he shook his head in a way that reassuringly said, "No." I adjusted his pillows, swabbed his mouth with water, and held his hand again. He settled down. My great nephew came over to see him. "Come in….it's ok. It's still your great granddaddy. He can hear you, but he can't talk," I said. He found some comfort in my words, stood next to me, and talked to my dad for a bit. In the early evening, my oldest nieces took over the evening shift. Before I left, my dad whispered, "Remember me." I thought, "How can I forget you? You're my dad." I didn't understand at the time it would be last time I saw him alive. My dad knew he was leaving that evening, but for some reason, despite my front-row seat with death, I expected to see him tomorrow morning at 6 am.

My younger niece called me at 5:30 the next morning sobbing, and I knew my dad had made his transition. Still clad in my pajamas, I rushed to my parents' house. In my rear-view mirror, I saw a siren-blazing ambulance and a fire truck. "Where are they going? Surely, they're not coming to my parents' house," I thought to myself. Under the care of Hospice, there's no need to call the two entities that save lives. Hospice will peacefully pronounce the death and call the funeral home. I met the ambulance and firemen to show them the Do Not Resuscitate order posted in the kitchen, which replaced postings for upcoming social engagements. Although the emergency medic and fireman weren't required attendees for my father's passing, I took solace in the fireman's observation of my dad. "He died peacefully," he said. The peaceful look on his face let me know he died without pain, which was so important given the insidious nature of pancreatic cancer. I kissed him on his forehead, just as I did every morning when he was alive. His forehead was cold, an alarming contrast to the warm, soft hand I had held the day before.

My family and neighbors came out of the woodwork and started reminiscing about fond memories. Although people surrounded me, I felt alone. My dad and I were on this journey together, and he was gone. *Now what?* Now, *I* was in a place between here and there — at the corner of Walk and Don't Walk.

What you can do…

If you are a caregiver, be sure to ask your nurses and counselors about the telltale signs of death. They will help you understand what is happening with your loved one. Despite your loved one's unresponsiveness, s/he can still hear you. Don't say anything hurtful or disregard his or her wishes. S/he can still hear, think, feel, and love.

Hours before death, understand your loved one may leave at any time. Be prepared to say goodbye every time you leave the bedside.

At the time of death, call Hospice, not 911. They will pronounce the death and call the funeral home. Hospice will also remove medications and medical supplies from your home.

If you are friends with a caregiver, be on standby and play your involvement by ear. This is a very intense time for caregivers — some want to be left alone, while others want company.

7

The Road Not Taken

Blazing Trails

My father's transition kicked off the usually flurry of funeral preparations. I was in charge of the program. My brother let me know the funeral home wanted a photo and a poem. Poem? What for? For the moment, I ignored this request and focused on scanning the photo my mom and dad had selected for the occasion. Two days went by, and the poem was due to the funeral home. I selected Robert Frost's, *The Road Not Taken,* one of my father's favorite poems. A friend offered to help me finish my toughest writing assignment, my dad's obituary. Afterwards, she said, "He was a real trailblazer. You must be so proud of him."

My dad was very involved in his community and blazed trails so the next generation could have opportunities. When faced with a challenge, he never asked, "Why?" Instead, he asked, "Why not?" As a result, he created opportunities where there were none. If a venture didn't work, he learned from it and tried something different. He used to say, "When one door closes, another one opens, and if you can't find a door, find a window!"

Two visions of my dad are etched in my memory. One memory is of him facing me with a wide smile and open arms, as if he was giving the world a big hug. His soundtrack is a snappy jazz tune, like Ramsey Lewis' "The In Crowd." My second vision represents my dad's twilight years; he walks peacefully away from this lifetime, keeping time to a mellow jazz tune, like "Mo Better Blues," by the Branford Marsalis Quartet. From where I am standing, he gets smaller on the horizon and eventually disappears from my physical world. I am honored to have held my dad's hand during that last mile, and I will never forget the precious moments I shared with him in this lifetime.

The funeral was packed with family, friends, neighbors, politicians, and even the membership guy from the golf club. All walks of life were represented, and I realized the array of people my dad had touched was far-reaching. The service included a fraternal hour of singing, a proclamation from Mecklenburg County in North Carolina, and a proclamation from the House of Congress for being a local and national Black political leader. Our Bishop delivered a passionate eulogy that made us laugh, cry, and contemplate our life purpose. The Army gave their salute and presented my mom with an American flag folded neatly into a perfect triangle. Afterwards, my friends and co-workers said repeatedly, "I never expected to be inspired at a funeral." They began to ask themselves, "What legacy will I leave behind?" I asked myself the same question. I thought about all those things on my bucket list. None of us really know how much time we have in this life; we just assume there *is* time.

Gifts and Lessons

For two years, I regretted not being physically present when my dad took his last breath. Finally, I realized my active presence and role as a primary caregiver made it possible for my dad to die peacefully. I *did* keep my promise to hold my dad's hand and drop him off at the pearly gates. It was then my mom's privilege, as his wife of 60 years, to take it from there – to tell him it was OK to go and to open the pearly gates for him. I was not supposed to be there for that intensely personal moment between my mom and dad.

The Hospice counselor told me at the beginning of the journey this experience would be a gift; however, I did not realize how many facets this gift would have. With Inky as my teacher, I learned to be fully present in the moment. I then gave my dad the gift of peace by walking with him on his difficult journey. My dad gave me the gift of time, a heightened sense of urgency to find my life purpose and follow my dreams. I recognized the gift of connection and community by allowing others to help my family and me. This renewed sense of connection and community planted seeds in my subconscious for the lessons I needed to *learn* in this lifetime.

Until my experiences with Inky and my dad, I ignored the healthy boundaries of self-care. I possessed a heightened sense of responsibility to follow through on most, if not all, of my commitments, whether large or small, reasonable or unreasonable. Caregiving stretched me beyond what was physically and emotionally possible, forcing me to retire my cape with my superpowers and ask for help. I learned helping others meant supporting not doing their work for them. I found new ways to support the people I loved without giving away all of myself.

These gifts and lessons have enabled me to get clearer about my life purpose and be fully present in each moment. The Universe, or God, will figure out the details; I just have to say, "Yes!" to the things I want to do in this life. Now, when I get to the corner of Walk and Don't Walk, I no longer assume I am lost. I take note of my surroundings, acknowledge the serendipities and synchronicities, and know the Universe will provide whatever I need to follow in my dad's footsteps and blaze my own trail.

What you can do…

If you are a caregiver, ask your friends and family for help with funeral arrangements. The funeral home will help with submitting the obituary to the local newspaper, filing paperwork for the life insurance policy, and logistics for the funeral.

Get help with the following items:

- Selecting a burial outfit for your loved one (including socks and underwear)
- Selecting a casket and tombstone
- Making decisions regarding the funeral arrangements
- Contributing to and proofreading the funeral program
- Deciding on transportation options provided by the funeral home
- Receiving visitors after the funeral, if desired
- Keeping a list of gifts and gestures for writing thank you notes
- Writing thank you notes

Be nice to yourself. Give yourself time and space to grieve. Surround yourself with loving people and remember to carve out time for introspection. If you have been a primary caregiver, allow yourself time to adjust to a new routine and setting.

Reacquaint yourself with your favorite activities or try new ones. Your house will feel empty without your loved one, but surprisingly the absence of medications and home health supplies will also make your surroundings feel empty.

If you are friends with a caregiver, offer to help in any way possible. Even the smallest of gestures means a lot. Offer to pick up dry cleaning, prepare a meal, or contribute financially for incidentals, such as stamps or meals. People grieve in different ways — some caregivers like company while others need solitude. Don't assume your friend wants to be left alone or have company, simply ask.

Avoid cliché platitudes and statements such as, "Your loved one is in a better place." This type of statement doesn't take away the pain your friend is feeling. Instead, it subtly suggests *how* a grieving person *should* feel about a loved one at this moment in time. An alternative is to offer your hope for peace during this difficult time.

The days get lonely for your caregiving friend after the funeral has taken place and others resume their normal routines. Check on your friend after the flurry of fried chicken, flowers, and cards has come and gone.

Friends and Caregivers' Guidebook

For each chapter in this book, you'll find a section here in the Friends and Caregivers' Guidebook. This section is intended to help you centralize all of your critical caregiving information, such as Hospice contacts, nurse schedules and volunteer information. Fill out each section as you go through the end of life stages with your loved one and then keep it in a handy place for you and others to reference.

You can also visit www.kymmotley.com/guidebook and enter the password "c@regiv1nG" to download a printable PDF version of this section.

1

Find Your Loved Ones and Meet Them There

Jot down information in preparation for and during your first doctor visit with your loved one:

Appointment date and time:

Doctor's name:

Doctor's office location:

Details from doctor visit:

Contact name and number for follow up questions:

2

Listen Intently, With Your Eyes, Ears and Heart

What does your loved one or caregiving friend need during this time? Take note of the top 5 things based on what you see, hear, or feel.

1.

2.

3.

4.

5.

Think of ways to incorporate these things into your caregiving routine or visits.

3

Send Love, No Matter What

Write a prayer or affirmation outlining what you want for your loved one. (Example: *I pray for my loved one to find peace during this difficult time.*)

Write a prayer or affirmation outlining what you want for your family members. Refer to this when your family members get on your nerves. It will remind you they, too, are hurting and searching for ways to deal with their impending loss.

4

Be Open to Hospice, Your New Best Friend

Write down your key contacts and routines to keep track of activities. Photocopy this section and complete it each week if home health schedules or medication changes occur.

Head Nurse: Counselor:

24/7 Hospice phone number:

Home Health Aid and Nurse Schedule: Write down the rotation schedule for home health aid and head nurse visits. Jot down any observations or questions you have for reference for the next visit.

	NAME	TIME	OBSERVATIONS/QUESTIONS
SUN			
MON			
TUES			
WED			
THURS			
FRI			
SAT			

Medication schedule: Track medications, dosage and dispensing times.

	AM	MIDDAY	EVENING	PM
SUN				
MON				
TUES				
WED				
THURS				
FRI				
SAT				

5

Ask For and Accept Help

Identify two people you trust and love to help you coordinate assistance from others:

Name: Phone number:

E-mail address:

Name: Phone number:

E-mail address:

Identify items you need help with:

Housekeeping:

Checking on your house:

Pet sitting:

Errands:

Groceries:

Meals:

Transportation:

Other:

Other:

6

The Final Days

Get help from your friends and family for the following tasks:

1. Schedule a family meeting with Hospice to prepare for your loved one's transition.
2. Create a call tree for announcing your loved one's death to avoid missing friends or close family.
3. After your loved one dies, work with the funeral home to file paperwork for the life insurance policy.
4. Write the obituary and select a photo of your loved one.
5. Work with the funeral home to gather information for the funeral program.
6. Gather clothes for the funeral home (don't forget underwear)!
7. Review the funeral program.
8. Make sure all family members know where and when to meet for the funeral.

7

The Road Not Taken

Life after losing a loved one is never the same. Be nice to yourself and ease into your next chapter. Take care of yourself by doing the following:

1. **Take advantage of counseling options through Hospice.** If you participate in group therapy, you will heal yourself and others.

2. **Give yourself permission to live with your loved ones' belongings for a while.** You don't have to give them away immediately. Consider giving items to family and close friends so they, too, can have a piece of your loved one.

3. **Consider giving back.** Support Hospice through a donation or volunteer in order to allow others to benefit from Hospice. If your loved one was passionate about an organization or cause, consider giving a donation in his/her honor. Doing so creates a legacy for your loved one and helps others in need.

About the Author

Throughout the years, Kym has tackled a myriad of creative endeavors including owning a woodshop, drawing, painting, mosaic tile, photography and jewelry. In the middle of creating her Spring 2010 jewelry collection, her kitty, Inky, and her father were both diagnosed with cancer. The jewelry stopped cold turkey but Kym kept a journal of her caregiving experiences. These journal entries turned into the book she wished she had during that time.

Kym currently lives in Manhattan, NY and finds inspiration in a good cup of coffee, food, art, and her orange kitty, Stinky. You can read about her artistic endeavors and adventures in New York City at www.kymmotley.com and www.dailymodernliving.com.

Made in United States
North Haven, CT
04 November 2026

21777545R00042